PENIS ENGLARGEMENT

Penis Growth: Bit by bit Penis Exercise Program, Augment Your Penis Normally (Penis Development Program, Jelqing, Male Enhancment, Penis Surgary, Greater Penis)

Doris R. Wheat

Table of Contents

CHAPTER 1

Penis enlargement

The human life system is an interesting subject that includes the investigation of the design and capability of the human body. It envelops different frameworks, each with its own interesting attributes and purposes. One of these frameworks is the conceptive framework, which is answerable for the production of new life. Inside the regenerative framework, there are particular contrasts between the male and female life structures. In this conversation, we will zero in on the male conceptive framework and investigate its fundamental parts and works.

The male conceptive framework is a complicated organization of organs, organs, and tissues that cooperate to create and convey sperm. It is basically answerable for the creation of male gametes (sperm cells) and the exchange of these phones to the female conceptive framework during sex. The essential organs of the male conceptive framework are the testicles, which are situated in the scrotum. The secretion of testosterone, a hormone that is essential to male development and fertility, and the production of sperm are both functions of the testes.

Notwithstanding the testicles, a few different designs make up the male regenerative framework. These incorporate the epididymis, vas deferens, fundamental vesicles, prostate organ, and penis. The epididymis is a looped tube situated behind every testis, where sperm mature and acquire the capacity to swim. The vas deferens is a strong cylinder that transports mature sperm from the epididymis to the urethra. Fluids that nourish and protect the sperm are produced by the prostate gland and the seminal vesicles. The penis, then again, is the outside organ liable for conveying sperm into the female conceptive framework during sex.

Understanding the male conceptive framework is fundamental for fathoming human propagation and richness. The perplexing interchange between the different organs and organs takes into account the formation of new life. By diving into the intricacies of the male regenerative framework, we gain a more profound appreciation for the wonders of human life structures and the inconceivable capacities of the human body.

The human life systems is a captivating field of study that looks at the design and elements of the human body. One explicit area of concentration inside this point is the life systems of the penis. The penis is a male conceptive organ engaged with sexual multiplication and pee. Understanding its life structures is fundamental for fathoming capabilities and potential medical problems might emerge.

The penis comprises of a few key designs. The shaft is the long, barrel shaped piece of the penis that reaches out from the base to the tip. It is made out of three barrel shaped collections of erectile tissue: two corpora cavernosa on the top and one corpus spongiosum under. The corpora cavernosa are liable for the penis' inflexibility during an erection, while the corpus spongiosum encompasses the urethra, taking into consideration the section of both pee and semen.

At the tip of the penis lies the glans, otherwise called the head. The glans is covered by a free overlay of skin called the prepuce, which can be taken out in a system called circumcision. The glans is profoundly delicate because of the presence of various sensitive spots, making it an essential piece of sexual joy. The opening at the tip of the glans is known as the urethral meatus, through which pee and semen pass.

There are many reasons why knowing the anatomy of the penis is important. It permits people to perceive any anomalies or potential medical problems that might emerge, like erectile brokenness or physically sent contaminations. Also, information on the penis' designs supports fathoming the mechanics of sex and regenerative wellbeing. By concentrating on the life structures of the penis, understudies can acquire a more profound comprehension of the male regenerative framework and its capabilities, adding to their general information on the human life systems. The study of the human body's structure and organization is a fascinating field known as human anatomy. One significant subtopic inside this field is the life systems of the testicles. The testicles are male regenerative organs that assume a critical part in the development of sperm and the discharge of testosterone. Situated inside the scrotum, the testicles are oval-formed and are suspended by a design called the spermatic rope.

The testicles are made out of a few layers that safeguard and backing their capability. The peripheral layer is known as the tunica vaginalis, which is a smooth film that covers the testicles and permits them to move uninhibitedly inside the scrotum. Underneath The human life systems is an entrancing subject that includes the investigation of the construction and capability of the human body. It includes a variety of systems, each with its own particular features and functions. One of these frameworks is the regenerative framework, which is answerable for the making of new life. Inside the regenerative framework, there are particular contrasts between the male and female life systems. In this conversation, we will zero in on the male conceptive framework and investigate its fundamental parts and works.

The male conceptive framework is a mind boggling organization of organs, organs, and tissues that cooperate to create and convey sperm. It is basically answerable for the creation of male gametes (sperm cells) and the exchange of these phones to the female conceptive framework during sex. The testes, which are found in the scrotum, are the primary organs of the male reproductive system. The secretion of testosterone, a hormone that is essential to male development and fertility, and the production of sperm are both functions of the testes.

Notwithstanding the testicles, a few different designs make up the male regenerative framework. These incorporate the epididymis, vas deferens, fundamental vesicles, prostate organ, and penis. The epididymis is a coiled tube behind each testis where mature sperm acquire swimming abilities. The vas deferens is a solid cylinder that transports mature sperm from the epididymis to the urethra. Fluids that nourish and protect the sperm are produced by the prostate gland and the seminal vesicles. The penis, then again, is the outer organ liable for conveying sperm into the female conceptive framework during sex.

Understanding human reproduction and fertility requires an understanding of the male reproductive system. The unpredictable exchange between the different organs and organs takes into account the production of new life. By digging into the intricacies of the male regenerative framework, we gain a more profound appreciation for the wonders of human life systems and the extraordinary capacities of the human body.

The human life systems is a captivating field of study that inspects the construction and elements of the human body. One explicit area of concentration inside this point is the life systems of the penis. The penis is a male reproductive organ that controls urination and sexual reproduction. Understanding its functions and potential health issues require an understanding of its anatomy.

The penis comprises of a few key designs. The long, oblong part of the penis that runs from the base to the tip is called the shaft. It is made out of three round and hollow groups of erectile tissue: two corpora cavernosa on the top and one corpus spongiosum under. The corpora cavernosa are liablc for thc penis' inflexibility during an erection, while the corpus spongiosum encompasses the urethra, taking into account the entry of both pee and semen.

At the tip of the penis lies the glans, otherwise called the head. The glans is covered by a free crease of skin called the prepuce, which can be eliminated in a strategy called circumcision. The glans is profoundly delicate because of the presence of various sensitive spots, making it a pivotal piece of sexual joy. The opening at the tip of the glans is known as the urethral meatus, through which pee and semen pass.

Understanding the life systems of the penis is significant in light of multiple factors. It permits people to perceive any anomalies or potential medical problems that might emerge, like erectile brokenness or physically sent contaminations. Moreover, information on the penis' designs supports fathoming the mechanics of sex and regenerative wellbeing. By concentrating on the life structures of the penis, understudies can acquire a more profound comprehension of the male conceptive framework and its capabilities, adding to their general information on the human life systems. The study of the human body's structure and organization is a fascinating field known as human anatomy. One significant subtopic inside this field is the life structures of the testicles. The male reproductive organs known as the testes are responsible for the production of sperm and the release of testosterone. Situated inside the scrotum, the testicles are oval-molded and are suspended by a design called the spermatic rope.

Chapter 2

Anatomy of the testes

Anatomy of the testes

The testes are protected and supported in their function by a number of layers. The furthest layer is known as the tunica vaginalis, which is a smooth film that covers the testicles and permits them to move unreservedly inside the scrotum. Under the regenerative framework gives knowledge into the intricacy and wonders of the human anatomy.ity and complexity of the human body.

Regular strategies allude to procedures or approaches that are gotten from nature and don't include the utilization of fake or engineered substances. These techniques are in many cases utilized in different parts of life, including medical care, agribusiness, and individual prosperity. The idea of regular techniques rotates around bridling the force of nature's assets to accomplish wanted results. By getting it and using normal strategies, people might possibly upgrade their general wellbeing, advance economical practices, and diminish their dependence on customary techniques.

In the domain of medical care, normal strategies center around utilizing regular cures and methods to forestall, treat, or oversee different ailments. This might include the utilization of home grown medication, dietary changes, exercise, and unwinding methods. Normal techniques focus on the body's inborn capacity to recuperate itself and expect to address the main driver of diseases instead of just mitigating side effects. Individuals may be able to reduce their exposure to harmful chemicals or side effects of conventional medical treatments by adopting natural methods.

In horticulture, normal techniques accentuate manageable and eco-accommodating practices for developing harvests and raising animals. By encouraging the use of organic fertilizers, crop rotation, and biological pest control, these strategies aim to work in harmony with nature. By keeping away from the utilization of manufactured pesticides and hereditarily changed life forms, normal techniques plan to safeguard the climate, save biodiversity, and advance better food creation. Moreover, regular cultivating rehearses frequently lead to greater produce that is liberated from compound buildups, which can help both the buyers and the actual ranchers.

With regards to individual prosperity, regular techniques envelop different regions like skincare, magnificence, and generally speaking taking care of oneself. Regular skincare items, for instance, are planned with fixings got from plants, spices, and natural oils, keeping away from brutal synthetic compounds that might be tracked down in ordinary beauty care products. Normal strategies likewise urge people to embrace solid way of life propensities, like standard activity, stress the board methods, and a decent eating regimen, to upgrade their physical and mental prosperity. Individuals can prioritize their overall health and minimize their environmental impact by embracing natural methods in their personal care routine.

All in all, regular strategies envelop many methods and approaches that draw motivation from nature. From medical services to agribusiness and individual prosperity, normal strategies focus on supportability, wellbeing, and the use of regular assets. By getting it and embracing normal techniques, people might possibly upgrade their personal satisfaction, advance ecological preservation, and lessen their dependence on fake or engineered substances. Understanding Penis Size:

Penis size is a point that frequently raises interest and worry among people, especially men. It is essential to take note of that there is an extensive variety of penis sizes, and varieties are entirely ordinary. Myths about penis size can be dispelled and healthy body image can be promoted by understanding the factors that affect penis size.

First and foremost, it is pivotal to recognize that hereditary qualities assume a critical part in deciding penis size. Like other actual qualities, for example, level and eye tone, penis size is to a not entirely set in stone by our qualities. It is acquired from our folks and can't be adjusted through regular strategies. People must comprehend that there is no "great" or "typical" size, as varieties are totally regular and ought not be a reason to worry.

Also, it is vital for address the misinterpretation that penis size straightforwardly relates with sexual execution or fulfillment. Many individuals erroneously accept that a bigger penis naturally means more noteworthy sexual delight for the two accomplices. However, compared to just penis size, research indicates that emotional connection, communication, and overall sexual compatibility are more closely linked to sexual satisfaction. It is critical to focus on open correspondence, common regard, and investigating various methods and positions to upgrade sexual encounters, as opposed to zeroing in exclusively on size.

Last but not least, it is essential to stress that body positivity and self-acceptance are essential when it comes to penis size. Society frequently sustains unreasonable norms, prompting weaknesses and low confidence. It is fundamental for people to comprehend that the size of their penis doesn't characterize their value or manliness. All things considered, zeroing in on by and large wellbeing, taking care of oneself, and keeping a positive self-perception is more significant for one's general prosperity and certainty.

All in all, understanding penis size includes recognizing the job of hereditary qualities, exposing misinterpretations about sexual execution, and advancing self-acknowledgment. By instructing ourselves as well as other people on these themes, we can encourage a more comprehensive and steady climate that values individual contrasts and advances body energy.

Natural methods for enlarging the penis are often viewed as a safer and less expensive alternative to surgery or medication, which is why many people are interested in learning more about them. One of the most normally suggested regular strategies for penis extension is through works out. These activities are intended to increment blood stream to the penile region, fortify the muscles, and possibly lead to expanded size over the long run.

Jelqing is one popular exercise for enlarging the penis. Jelqing includes utilizing a hand-over-hand movement to back rub and stretch the penis. The reason for this exercise is to increment blood course and grow the penile tissues, which might bring about a more drawn out and thicker penis. It is essential to note that jelqing should be carried out with extreme caution and under the supervision of a professional, as regenerative framework gives knowledge into the intricacy and wonders of the human anatomy.ity and complexity of the human body.

Regular strategies allude to procedures or approaches that are gotten from nature and don't include the utilization of fake or engineered substances. These techniques are in many cases utilized in different parts of life, including medical care, agribusiness, and individual prosperity. The idea of regular techniques rotates around bridling the force of nature's assets to accomplish wanted results. By getting it and using normal strategies, people might possibly upgrade their general wellbeing, advance economical practices, and diminish their dependence on customary techniques.

In the domain of medical care, normal strategies center around utilizing regular cures and methods to forestall, treat, or oversee different ailments. This might include the utilization of home grown medication, dietary changes, exercise, and unwinding methods. Normal techniques focus on the body's inborn capacity to recuperate itself and expect to address the main driver of diseases instead of just mitigating side effects. Individuals may be able to reduce their exposure to harmful chemicals or side effects of conventional medical treatments by adopting natural methods.

In horticulture, normal techniques accentuate manageable and eco-accommodating practices for developing harvests and raising animals. By encouraging the use of organic fertilizers, crop rotation, and biological pest control, these strategies aim to work in harmony with nature. By keeping away from the utilization of manufactured pesticides and hereditarily changed life forms, normal techniques plan to safeguard the climate, save biodiversity, and advance better food creation. Moreover, regular cultivating rehearses frequently lead to greater produce that is liberated from compound buildups, which can help both the buyers and the actual ranchers.

With regards to individual prosperity, regular techniques envelop different regions like skincare, magnificence, and generally speaking taking care of oneself. Regular skincare items, for instance, are planned with fixings got from plants, spices, and natural oils, keeping away from brutal synthetic compounds that might be tracked down in ordinary beauty care products. Normal strategies likewise urge people to embrace solid way of life propensities, like standard activity, stress the board methods, and a decent eating regimen, to upgrade their physical and mental prosperity. Individuals can prioritize their overall health and minimize their environmental impact by embracing natural methods in their personal care routine.

All in all, regular strategies envelop many methods and approaches that draw motivation from nature. From medical services to agribusiness and individual prosperity, normal strategies focus on supportability, wellbeing, and the use of regular assets. By getting it and embracing normal techniques, people might possibly upgrade their personal satisfaction, advance ecological preservation, and lessen their dependence on fake or engineered substances.

Chapter 3

Understanding Penis Size

Penis size is a point that frequently raises interest and worry among people, especially men. It is essential to take note of that there is an extensive variety of penis sizes, and varieties are entirely ordinary. Myths about penis size can be dispelled and healthy body image can be promoted by understanding the factors that affect penis size.

First and foremost, it is pivotal to recognize that hereditary qualities assume a critical part in deciding penis size. Like other actual qualities, for example, level and eye tone, penis size is to a not entirely set in stone by our qualities. It is acquired from our folks and can't be adjusted through regular strategies. People must comprehend that there is no "great" or "typical" size, as varieties are totally regular and ought not be a reason to worry.

Also, it is vital for address the misinterpretation that penis size straightforwardly relates with sexual execution or fulfillment. Many individuals erroneously accept that a bigger penis naturally means more noteworthy sexual delight for the two accomplices.

However, compared to just penis size, research indicates that emotional connection, communication, and overall sexual compatibility are more closely linked to sexual satisfaction. It is critical to focus on open correspondence, common regard, and investigating various methods and positions to upgrade sexual encounters, as opposed to zeroing in exclusively on size.

Last but not least, it is essential to stress that body positivity and self-acceptance are essential when it comes to penis size. Society frequently sustains unreasonable norms, prompting weaknesses and low confidence. It is fundamental for people to comprehend that the size of their penis doesn't characterize their value or manliness. All things considered, zeroing in on by and large wellbeing, taking care of oneself, and keeping a positive self-perception is more significant for one's general prosperity and certainty.

All in all, understanding penis size includes recognizing the job of hereditary qualities, exposing misinterpretations about sexual execution, and advancing self-acknowledgment. By instructing ourselves as well as other people on these themes, we can encourage a more comprehensive and steady climate that values individual contrasts and advances body energy.

Natural methods for enlarging the penis are often viewed as a safer and less expensive alternative to surgery or medication, which is why many people are interested in learning more about them. One of the most normally suggested regular stratcgics for pcnis cxtcnsion is through works out. These activities are intended to increment blood stream to the penile region, fortify the muscles, and possibly lead to expanded size over the long run.

Jelqing is one popular exercise for enlarging the penis. Jelqing includes utilizing a hand-over-hand movement to back rub and stretch the penis. The reason for this exercise is to increment blood course and grow the penile tissues, which might bring about a more drawn out and thicker penis. It is vital to take note of that jelqing ought to be finished with alert and under the direction of an expert, as mistaken procedure or exorbitant power might cause injury.

One more activity that is frequently proposed for penis augmentation is called kegel works out. Kegel practices are ordinarily connected with reinforcing the pelvic floor muscles, yet they can likewise have benefits for penis wellbeing. The muscles that control urination and ejaculation are contracted and relaxed during these exercises. People may experience increased size, stronger erections, and improved blood flow to the penis if they perform kegel exercises on a regular basis.

Generally, practices for penis broadening are a characteristic technique that a few people might see as supportive. In any case, it is vital to move toward these strategies with alert and talk with a medical services proficient or a trustworthy source prior to beginning any work-out everyday practice. It is additionally vital to have sensible assumptions, as results might shift and critical size changes may not be attainable through practices alone. Home grown cures have been utilized for a really long time to treat different ailments, and one region where they are frequently pursued is in penis extension. Numerous men want a bigger penis in light of multiple factors, like expanded certainty or worked on sexual execution. While there is a large number of home grown cures accessible, understanding their viability and potential risks is significant.

One well known home grown solution for penis broadening is ginkgo biloba. It is thought that this herb increases blood flow, which may assist in getting and maintaining an erection. It is likewise remembered to build the size of vcins, bringing about a bigger penis. However, it is essential to note that there are few scientific studies on the efficacy of ginkgo biloba for enlarging the penis. Thusly, it is vital to move toward this cure with alert and talk with a medical services proficient prior to attempting it.

One more natural cure that is much of the time referenced with regards to penis amplification is Panax ginseng. This herb has been shown to increase libido and sexual function. A few investigations propose that it might likewise decidedly affect penis size. In any case, like ginkgo biloba, the logical proof supporting the utilization of Panax ginseng for penis broadening isn't broad. It is prudent to examine its utilization with a medical care supplier to guarantee security and viability.

Taking everything into account, natural solutions for penis amplification have been pursued by numerous people for a really long time. Even though some herbs, like ginkgo biloba and Panax ginseng, have traditionally been used for this purpose, it's important to use them with caution and talk to a doctor before doing so. Logical proof with respect to their viability and security is restricted, so it is vital to settle on informed choices and focus on personalNatural strategies allude to the utilization of non-engineered or natural ways to deal with address different wellbeing concerns. While these strategies are frequently viewed as protected and have been utilized for quite a long time, understudies must comprehend the potential dangers related with their utilization. One significant advantage of normal strategies is that they regularly have less secondary effects contrasted with drug drugs. This is due to the fact that natural treatments frequently make use of plants, herbs, or other natural substances that are kind to the body. In any case, it is critical to take note of that on the grounds that a technique is regular doesn't naturally mean it is ok for everybody. A few people might have sensitivities or aversions to specific normal substances, which can prompt unfriendly responses. Subsequently, it is fundamental to talk with a medical care proficient prior to attempting any normal strategy to guarantee its security and propriety for individual conditions.

Chapter 4

Pontential side effect penis enlargement method

One more security thought with regards to normal techniques is the potential for drug collaborations. Even though natural remedies can be effective on their own, they can sometimes interact with prescription medications, which can either make the medication less effective or cause unexpected side effects. For instance, certain spices or enhancements might increment or decline the impacts of blood-diminishing drugs, prompting an expanded gamble of draining or coagulating. In this manner, it is critical for people to illuminate their medical services suppliers about any regular cures they are utilizing or wanting to use, to stay away from any possible dangers or entanglements.

Last but not least, it's critical to keep in mind that natural treatments might not always be enough to treat some health issues. While they can be compelling for gentle or constant circumstances, a few intense or serious sicknesses might require more quick and concentrated clinical intercession. It is fundamental for understudies to comprehend that regular strategies ought not be viewed as a substitute for clinical consideration, particularly in situations of emergency Postponing or staying away from clinical treatment for normal cures can be perilous and possibly dangerous. Accordingly, it is crucial to keep up with open correspondence with medical care experts and to look for their direction when required, to guarantee the security and prosperity of oneself or others. Worries about penis size are a typical issue among men that can essentially affect their confidence and generally speaking prosperity. Numerous people might feel unreliable or disappointed with the size of their penis, prompting insecurities or even uneasiness. It is vital to comprehend that worries about penis size can originate from different variables, including cultural assumptions, media impact, or even private encounters. Be that as it may, it is vital to move toward this theme with responsiveness and spotlight on advancing solid survival techniques and options.

One method for dealing with stress for people worried about penis size is instruction and mindfulness. By looking into the typical size scope of penises and understanding that there is critical variety among men, people can acquire a more reasonable viewpoint. It is fundamental to stress that penis size doesn't decide one's worth or capacity to physically fulfill an accomplice. Open communication and discussion about sexual satisfaction can help people realize that a satisfying sexual experience requires more than just a large penis.

Another survival technique is to zero in on self-acknowledgment and confidence.

Concerns about penis size can be alleviated by encouraging people to accept their bodies as they are and to appreciate the unique qualities they possess. Advancing positive self-perception and confidence can be accomplished through practices like taking care of oneself, participating in proactive tasks, and looking for proficient help when required. Empowering people to see the value in their general wellbeing and prospcrity as opposed to focusing exclusively on penis size can assist with moving their concentration to a more comprehensive viewpoint.

Last but not least, it is essential to acknowledge that seeking assistance from professionals or other reputable individuals can be extremely beneficial. Empowering people to examine their interests with a medical services supplier or an emotional wellness expert can give them the vital direction and instruments to successfully adapt to their concerns. These experts can assist people with creating sound survival techniques, challenge pessimistic considerations, and offer help in the meantime. Advancing an open and non-critical climate where people can look for help unafraid of disgrace is fundamental for tending to worries about penis size successfully. Understanding and surveying worries about penis size is a significant part of tending to self-perception and confidence issues in people. Many individuals, especially men, may encounter uneasiness or stress over the size of their penis. Recognizing that people's penis sizes vary widely and that the concept of an "ideal" sizc is subjcctive and influenced by societal and cultural factors is essential. By understanding the variables that add to worries about penis size, people can foster methods for dealing with especially difficult times to address these worries and further develop their general prosperity.

One method for understanding worries about penis size is to investigate the impact of media and cultural assumptions. The media frequently depicts a restricted and unreasonable norm of magnificence, including a specific size and state of the penis. This can lead people to contrast themselves with these unreasonable principles and feel deficient. Concerns about penis size can also be exacerbated by societal norms and stereotypes about men's masculinity. Understanding these outer impacts can assist people with perceiving that their interests might be unwarranted or misrepresented, and permit them to challenge these cultural tensions.

Surveying worries about penis size includes recognizing the close to home effect it might have on people. Anxiety, depression, and low self-esteem are all possible side effects for many people who are concerned about their penis size. It is essential to approve these sentiments and offer help to the people who are battling with these worries. Looking for proficient assistance, like treatment or guiding, can be helpful in resolving these intense subject matters. Furthermore, transparent correspondence with believed accomplices or companions can assist people with acquiring point of view and consolation.

Creating ways of dealing with hardship or stress is pivotal in overseeing worries about penis size. Focusing on overall body acceptance and self-love is one effective strategy. By perceiving and valuing the novel characteristics and qualities of their whole body, people can move their concentrate away from the size of their penis. Participating in certain self-talk and rethinking negative contemplations can likewise help in building fearlessness. It is additionally critical to recall that sexual fulfillment and closeness are not set in stone by penis size. Creating solid correspondence and profound associations with accomplices can enormously upgrade sexual encounters. Investigating elective types of sexual delight and closeness, for example, oral sex or the utilization of sex toys, can likewise assist people with feeling more sure and fulfilled in their sexual connections.

All in all, understanding and evaluating worries about penis size is urgent for people battling with self-perception and confidence issues. By perceiving the impact of media and cultural assumptions, people can challenge unreasonable principles and foster a more certain self-perception. In order to address the underlying emotional issues, it is essential to evaluate the emotional impact of these worries and, if necessary, seek professional assistance. In conclusion, creating survival methods, like zeroing in on generally speaking body acknowledgment and investigating elective types of sexual delight, can assist people with working on their fearlessness and by and large prosperity. Worries about penis size can be a wellspring of trouble for some people, influencing their confidence and by and large prosperity. It is vital to perceive that penis size isn't the main element that adds to sexual satisfaction and delight. There are different elective survival methods that people can utilize to address their interests and work on their sexual encounters.

One elective way of dealing with hardship or stress is correspondence. Transparently examining worries about penis size with an accomplice can assist with mitigating uneasiness and establish a steady climate. Powerful correspondence can include communicating one's frailties, looking for consolation, and talking about what the two accomplices view as pleasurable. By discussing their thoughts and wants, people can cultivate a more profound comprehension and association, prompting upgraded sexual fulfillment.

Another survival method is zeroing in on joy as opposed to measure. It is fundamental to recollect that sexual joy isn't exclusively reliant upon penis size yet is a perplexing exchange of physical, close to home, and mental perspectives. Taking part in exercises that focus on generally speaking delight, like foreplay, oral sex, or utilizing sex toys, can assist with moving the concentrate away from size and towards the investigation of various sensations and joy zones. By extending one's sexual collection, people can find better approaches to encounter delight and upgrade their sexual fulfillment.

Finally, looking for proficient assist with canning be an important survival technique for people battling with worries about penis size. Counseling a medical services proficient or a specialist who spends significant time in sexual wellbeing can give direction and backing. These experts can offer proof based data, address concerns, and give customized techniques to work on generally sexual prosperity. They can assist people with fostering a better outlook, challenge pessimistic convictions, and

investigate strategies to improve
joy and closeness.

Chapter 5

Safety concerns with medical procedures for penis enlargement

All in all, worries about penis size can essentially affect people's confidence and sexual fulfillment. In any case, elective survival methods can assist people with tending to these worries and further develop their general prosperity. By encouraging open correspondence, zeroing in on joy as opposed to measure, and looking for proficient assistance, people can foster a better mentality and upgrade their sexual encounters. Worries about penis size can be a critical wellspring of pain for some people, influencing their confidence, certainty, and generally personal satisfaction. In any case, it is fundamental to comprehend that there are guiding and treatment choices accessible to address these worries and assist people with adapting to their sentiments. One such choice is individual guiding, where a prepared specialist can give a protected and steady climate to investigate and deal with these worries. During individual directing meetings, people can talk about their sentiments, fears, and frailties connected with penis size, and the specialist can offer direction, consolation, and survival methods to successfully deal with these worries.

Bunch treatment is another restorative choice that can be gainful for people managing worries about penis size. Joining a gathering of people who share comparative worries can give a feeling of approval and backing, as members can straightforwardly examine their encounters and sentiments unafraid of judgment. Bunch treatment meetings frequently include sharing individual stories, investigating hidden convictions and presumptions about manliness and self-esteem, and gaining from other people who have effectively adapted to comparative worries. Through bunch treatment, people can acquire another viewpoint, improve their self-acknowledgment, and foster solid survival techniques.

As well as guiding and treatment, there are other survival methods that people can use to oversee worries about penis size. One such systcm is instruction and self-strengthening. By investigating and understanding the extensive variety of ordinary penis sizes, people can challenge ridiculous cultural guidelines and foster a more practical and positive view of themselves. Participating in taking care of oneself exercises, like activity, reflection, and care, can likewise be useful in diminishing pressure and upgrading in general prosperity. Moreover, keeping up with transparent correspondence with an accomplice about these worries can encourage grasping, acknowledgment, and backing, at last fortifying the relationship.

It is critical to recollect that worries about penis size are substantial and can altogether affect a person's close to home and mental prosperity. Notwithstanding, looking for proficient assist through advising and treatment choices with canning offer the fundamental help and direction to successfully address these worries. By using survival methods and fostering a more certain mentality, people can figure out how to acknowledge and embrace their bodies, prompting worked on confidence and a better identity. Numerous people might encounter worrics about their penis size, which can affect their confidence, certainty, and generally speaking prosperity. It is critical to comprehend that penis size shifts among people, and what makes the biggest difference is the means by which one feels about their own body. There are different way of life changes and survival techniques that can assist people with conquering their interests in regards to penis size.

Right off the bat, embracing a sound way of life can emphatically affect one's general prosperity and fearlessness. Taking part in ordinary actual activity works on actual wellbeing as well as lifts confidence. Exercise can assist people with feeling more great in their own bodies and diminish deep-seated insecurities connected with penis size. Moreover, keeping a decent eating routine and remaining hydrated can add to by and large wellbeing and prosperity, which thusly can work on self-insight and certainty.

Besides, it is vital for people to zero in on self-acknowledgment and confidence. Tolerating and embracing oneself overall, as opposed to focusing on one explicit part of the body, is essential for building certainty and defeating worries about penis size. Taking part in exercises that advance taking care of oneself and fearlessness, for example, rehearsing care, pondering, or taking part in leisure activities and interests, can assist people with fostering a positive self-perception and adapt to worries about penis size.

Finally, looking for help from confided in people, like companions, family, or a specialist, can give important direction and viewpoint. Discussing concerns and weaknesses with somebody who can offer help and understanding can be extraordinarily useful. A specialist or instructor can likewise give proficient direction and devices to adapting to self-perception concerns. Moreover, joining support gatherings or online networks where people can share encounters and guidance can make a feeling of fortitude and assist people with acknowledging they are in good company in their interests.

All in all, worries about penis size can be upsetting for people, however there are different way of life changes and survival methods that can assist with defeating these worries. Embracing a solid way of life, zeroing in on self-acknowledgment and self esteem, and looking for help from believed people are exceedingly significant stages in working on confidence and prosperity. It is essential to recollect that everybody's body is one of a kind, and what makes the biggest difference is the manner by which one feels about themselves, as opposed to adjusting to cultural goals.